Harnessing Nature's Remedies in Essential Oil

A Comprehensive Guide to Essential Oils' Benefit for Healthy Living

By

Tatiana Andres

Copyright ©2024 Tatiana Andres,

All rights reserved

Disclaimer

The information contained in this book and its contents are mainly for educational purposes, and may not be taken as or seen as an alternative to Medical advice.

As compiled by Tatiana Andres

Edited by Ahaotu Franklin Ndubuisi

Table of Contents

Introduction

Step into the vast world of essential oils with this all-encompassing guide, unlocking nature's potent remedies. As your trusted companion, this handbook reveals the therapeutic, aromatic, and holistic potential of essential oils.

Join me on a journey through the essence of natural healing. Explore lavender's calming embrace, the invigorating zest of citrus oils, and the revitalizing power of peppermint. Let's discover how the tea tree defends and how eucalyptus clears the senses.

This comprehensive guide isn't just a list of oils—it's a treasure trove of knowledge. I'll guide you through the art of extraction, unravel the science behind their potency, and illuminate the meticulous processes that yield these precious essences. We'll delve into sourcing, quality assessment, and ethical practices in the world of essential oils.

Let's delve into practical applications together. Whether it's infusing tranquillity into your living space, crafting skincare medicines, or enhancing culinary creations, we'll harness the therapeutic potential in every drop. Together, we'll find solutions for everyday ailments, wellness routines, and emotional balance.

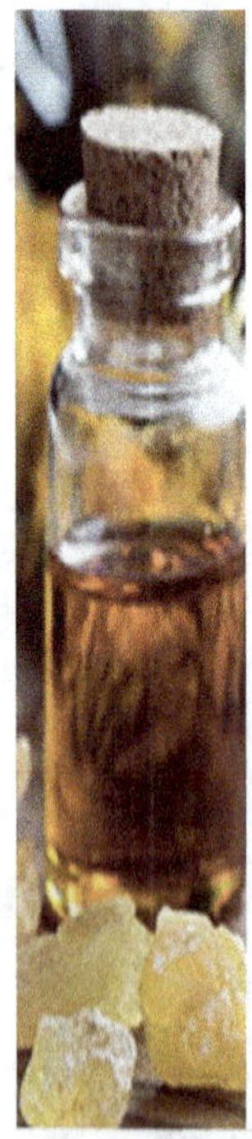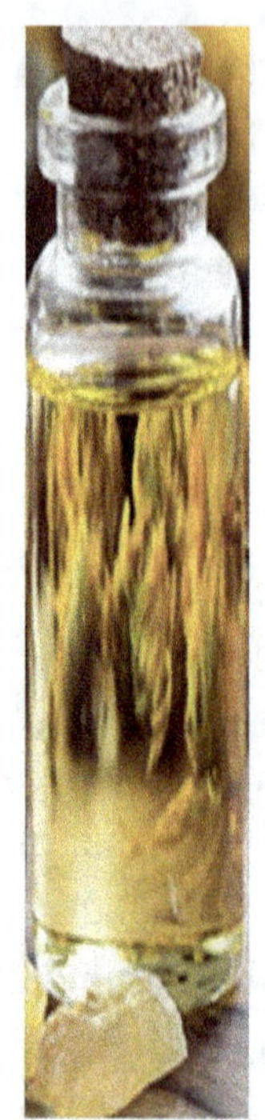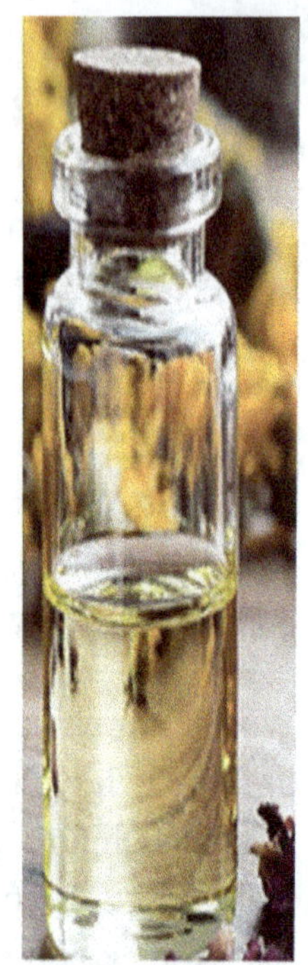

Within these pages, expert insights, detailed oil profiles, safety guidelines, and DIY recipes await. We'll immerse ourselves in the world of aromatherapy, holistic healing, and natural remedies.

Join me in this world of essential oils. Together, let's unlock the power of nature, one drop at a time.

Chapter 1

Essential Oils, Definition and Origin

Essential oils are highly concentrated natural extracts from plants, like flowers, leaves, or roots. They're packed with the special stuff that gives plants their scent and unique properties. These oils can be used in things like aromatherapy, skincare, or even cleaning because they have cool abilities to help you relax, feel better, or smell amazing. Just a tiny bit can go a long way because they're super potent.

Essential oils have been around for a super long time—like ancient civilization. People from way back, like the Egyptians, Greeks, and even the Chinese, used these oils for all sorts of things. These include medicines, perfumes, and even religious ceremonies. They've been a part of human life for thousands of years, and people have always known they're exceptional.

Cultural Use of essential oils

Essential oils have an ancient origin, dating back thousands of years. They were first discovered through processes like distillation, where people figured out how to extract these powerful, fragrant oils from plants like flowers, leaves, and roots. Early civilizations like the Egyptians, Greeks, and Chinese are recorded as among the first to use these oils for various purposes which I have mentioned to be as medicine, perfumes, and other religious or cultural rituals. Over time, this knowledge and use of essential oils spread across different cultures, becoming an essential part of traditional remedies and daily life.

The artistic use of essential oils is fascinating. For centuries, different cultures around the world have embraced it. In **ancient Egypt**, essential oils were highly prized and used in **religious ceremonies**, for **skin care**, and even in the **embalming** process for **mummies**.

The **Greeks** also valued essential oils, using them for their **medicinal properties** and in their **bathhouses** for **relaxation**.

In **Asia**, particularly in countries like **China** and **India**, essential oils were integrated into **traditional medicine practices** like **Ayurveda** and Traditional Chinese Medicine, where they were believed to have healing properties for the **body** and **mind**.

In more recent times, essential oils have found their way into various cultural practices worldwide, used mainly in **aromatherapy** for relaxation and stress relief and incorporated into skincare routines for their **natural benefits.**

The Usefulness of Essential Oil in Modern Wellness

Essential oils have become a big deal in modern wellness for some really good reasons. They're like nature's superheroes, packed with all these amazing properties that can help us feel better physically and emotionally.

Most people remember these oils when they want to relax, de-stress, and even boost moods. You know that calm feeling you get when you catch a whiff of a nice-smelling flower? That's the kind of thing essential oils do.

Plus, they're natural and very useful in making our skin happy and healthy. Some essential oils have properties that can soothe skin or make it super soft.

People are also finding ways to use these oils to tackle everyday issues, like using them in cleaning products to make things smell fresh without using harsh chemicals.

Examples of Essential Oils

There are tons of essential oils out there, each with its own special powers. I would discuss some of them in no particular other but starting with the most popular ones and their uses like:-

1. Lavender:- This one's like a chill pill in a bottle. It helps you relax and can even help you sleep better.

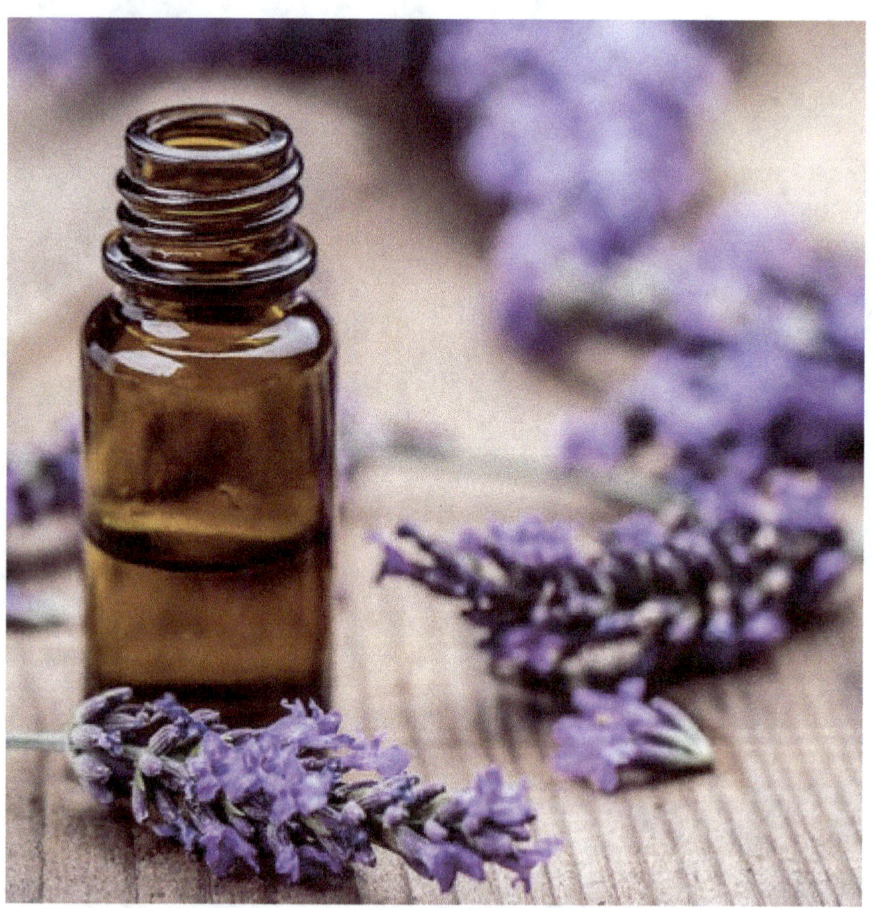

2. Peppermint:- It's like a burst of freshness. Peppermint oil can wake you up and make you feel more alert.

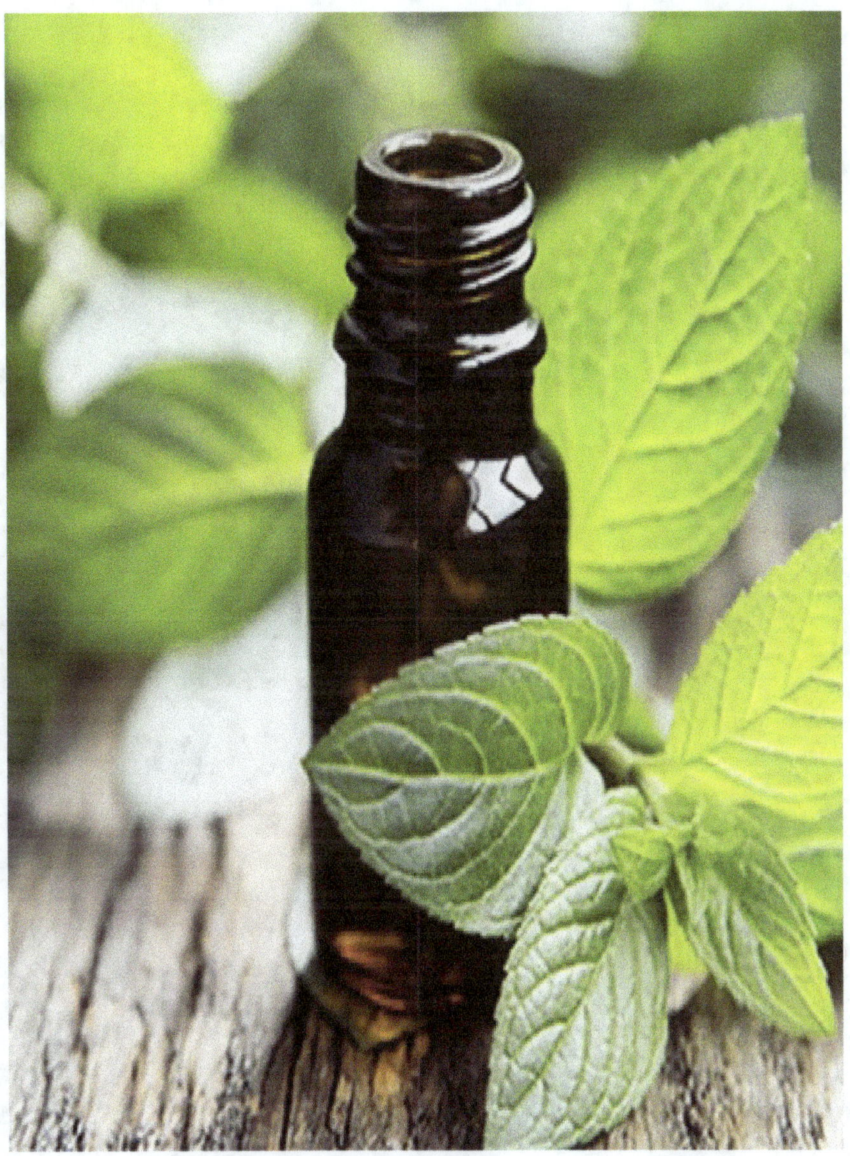

3. Tea Tree:- This oil is like a superhero for your skin. It can help fight off blemishes and keep your skin feeling clean.

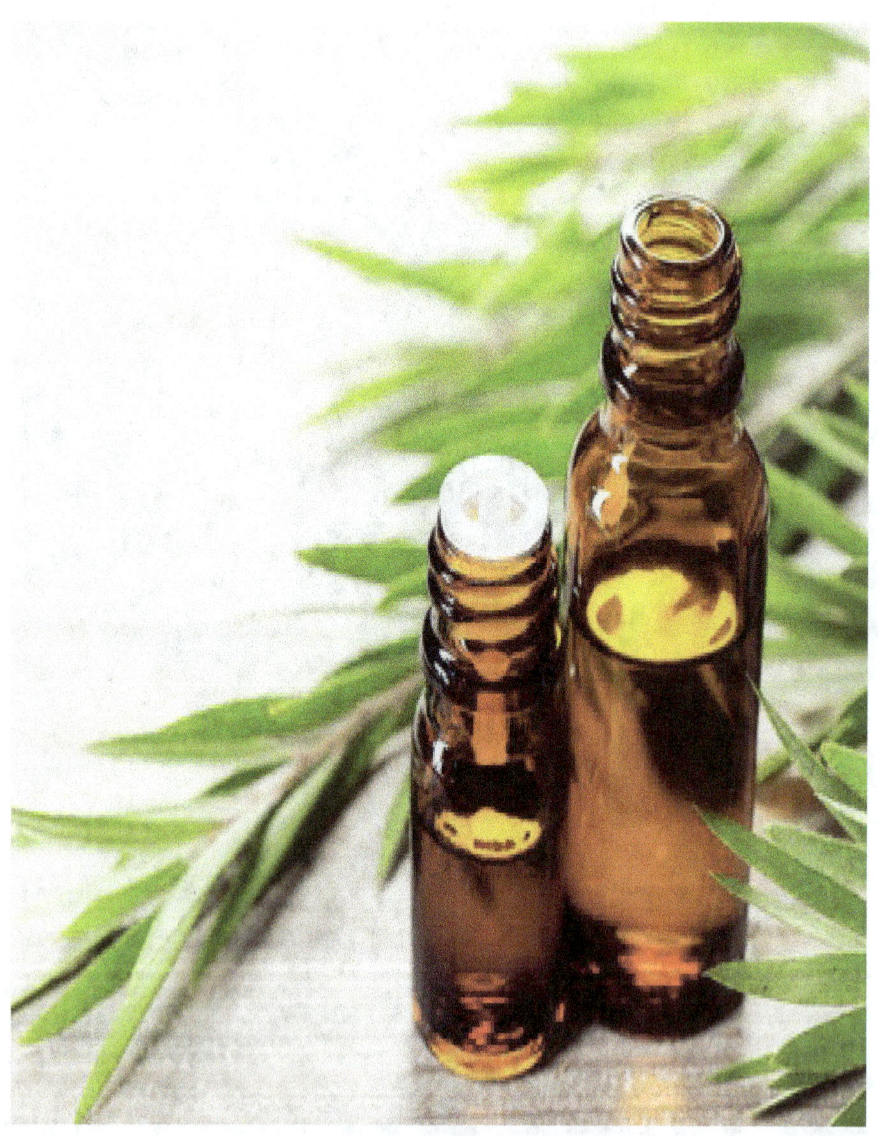

4. Eucalyptus:- Have you ever smelled it when you have a stuffy nose? That's because eucalyptus can clear your airways and help you breathe better.

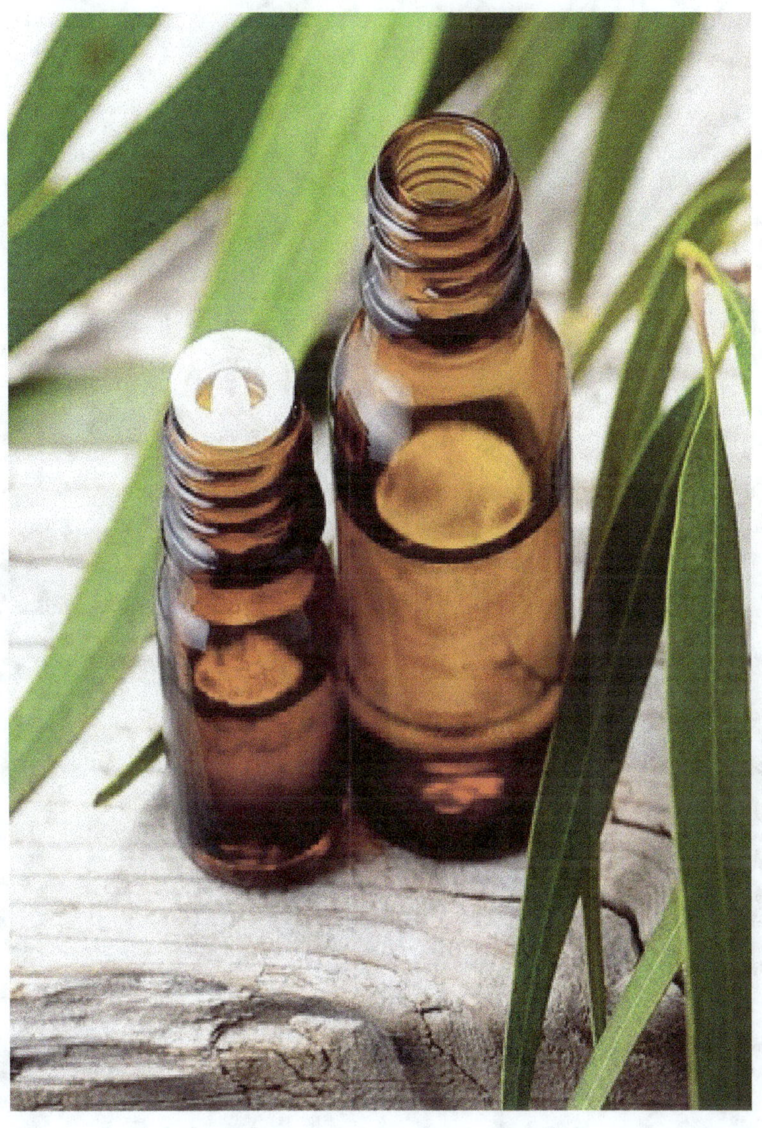

5. Lemon:- It's like sunshine in a bottle. Lemon oil smells fresh and can boost your mood.

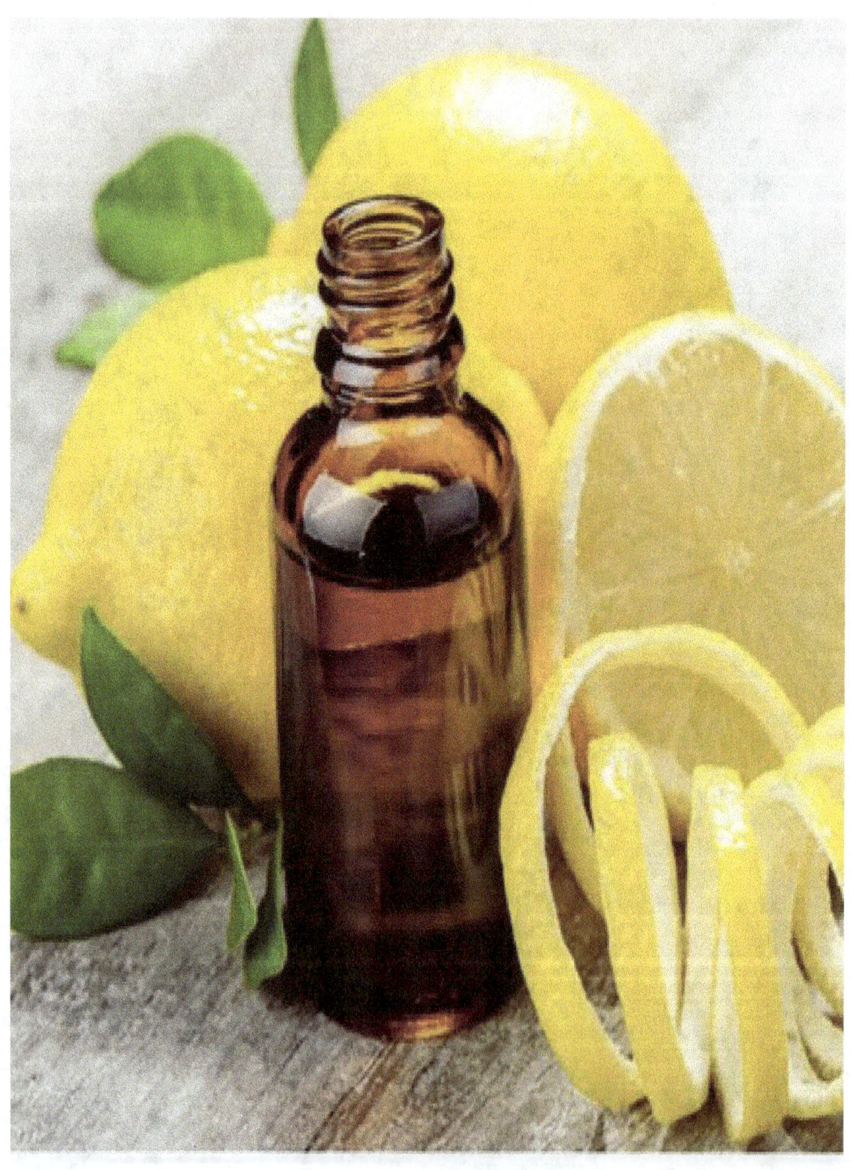

6. Chamomile:- This oil is like a cosy blanket. It's calming and can help you unwind after a long day.

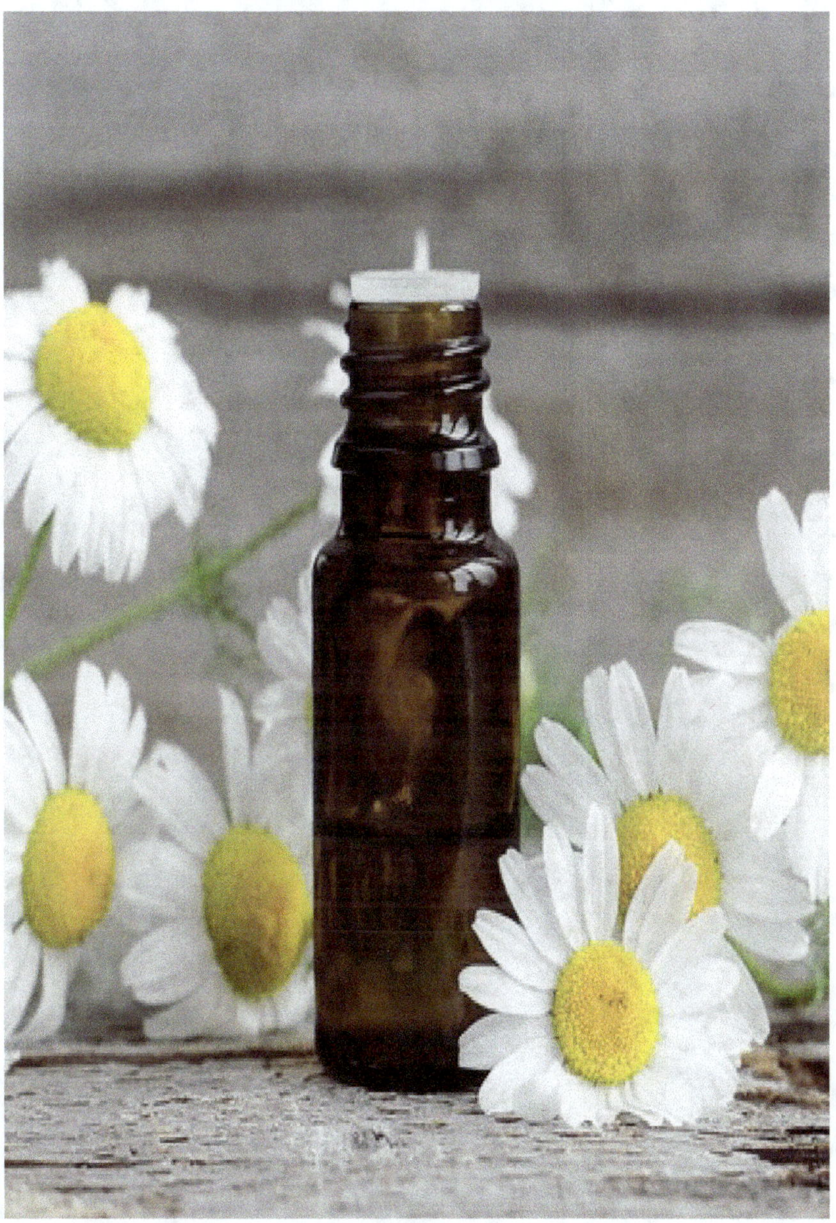

7. Frankincense:- Known for its calming properties, it's great for relaxation and can even help with focus during meditation.

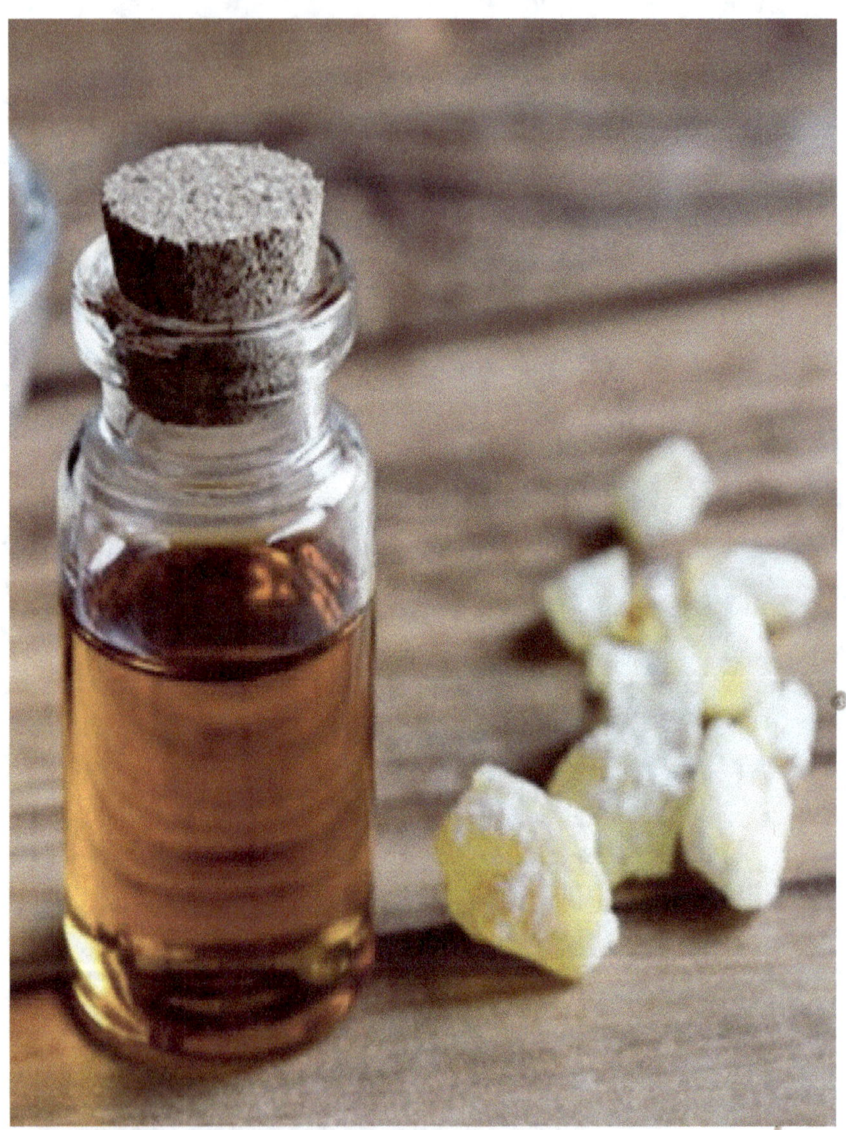

8. Rosemary:- A fantastic pick-me-up. Rosemary oil can boost your energy levels and help with mental clarity.

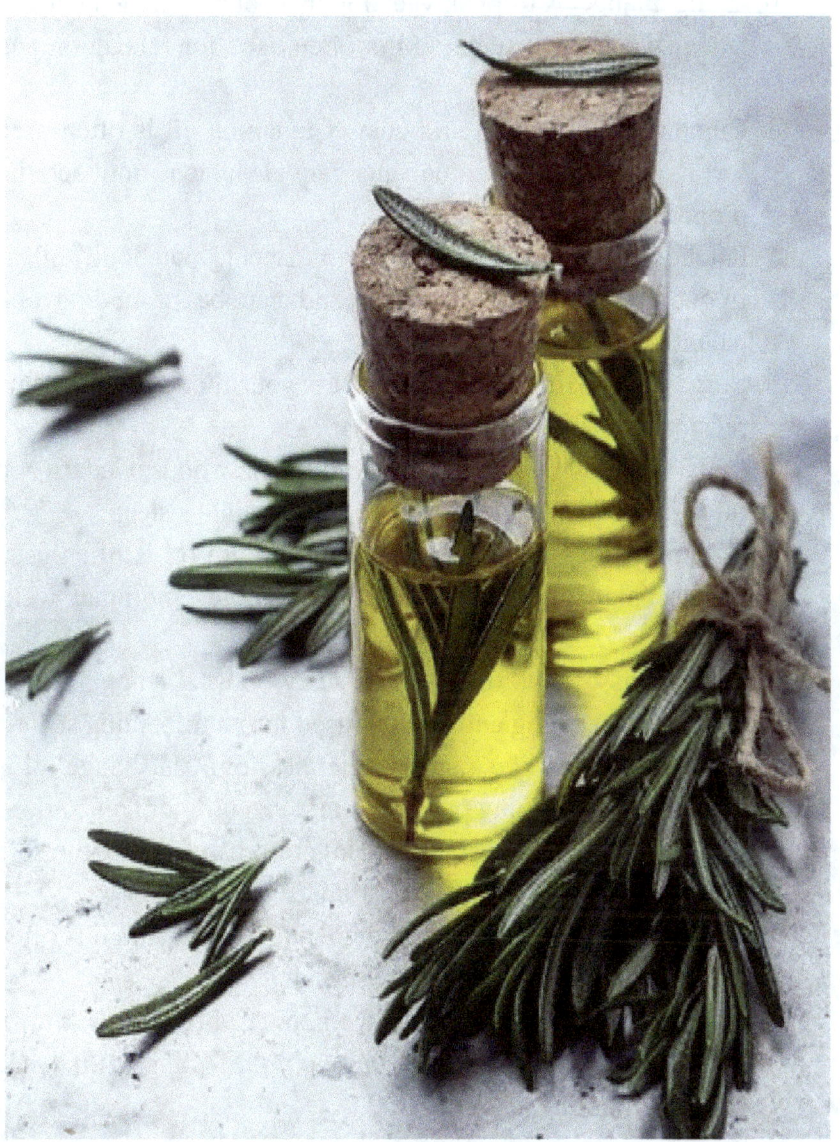

9. Sandalwood:- Sandalwood is more of a stress buster. The oil is great for calming nerves and promoting a sense of peace.
10. Ylang Ylang:- A tropical vacation in a bottle. Ylang Ylang oil has a sweet floral scent and is often used for relaxation and mood enhancement.
11. Cinnamon:- It's warm and cosy. Cinnamon oil is often used for its comforting aroma and can also have antibacterial properties.
12. Patchouli:- Known for its earthy scent, patchouli oil is frequently used for relaxation and can be grounding and balancing.
13. Bergamot:- Bergamot oil can uplift your mood and promote relaxation.
14. Cedarwood:- This one's like a walk in the woods. Cedarwood oil is calming and can help with a good night's sleep.
15. Geranium:- It's like a floral hug. Geranium oil is often used for its balancing effects and can promote emotional well-being.
16. Lemongrass:- This oil is like a zesty boost. Lemongrass oil can be invigorating and is often used for its refreshing scent.
17. Clary Sage:- It's like a stress relief session. Clary Sage oil is known for its calming properties and can promote relaxation.
18. Ginger:- This one's warming. Ginger oil can help soothe sore muscles and might aid in digestion.
19. Marjoram:- This oil is like a gentle hug. Marjoram oil is often used for relaxation and to ease muscle tension.
20. Cypress:- It's like a breath of fresh air. Cypress oil is known for its refreshing scent and can help with feelings of balance and grounding.

21. Juniper Berry:- Often equated to a forest adventure. Juniper Berry oil can have a fresh, woodsy scent and might support healthy skin.
22. Neroli:- Think about a bouquet of flowers. Neroli oil has a lovely floral aroma and is often used to promote relaxation and reduce stress.
23. Helichrysum:- This oil is people's favourite healing balm. Helichrysum oil is valued for its potential skin benefits and might help with minor skin irritations.
24. Black Pepper:- Valued it as a spicy surprise. Black Pepper oil can have a warm, stimulating effect and might support circulation.
25. Basil:- Gives us that typical burst of freshness. Basil oil is often used for its uplifting aroma and might help with focus and mental clarity.
26. Fennel:- Appreciated for a sweet treat. Fennel oil can have a sweet, licorice-like scent and might aid in digestion.
27. Tangerine:- It's another typical sunshine in a bottle. Tangerine oil has a bright, citrusy scent and can promote a cheerful atmosphere.
28. Thyme:- Many say this oil is an herbal powerhouse. Thyme oil is known for its potential antibacterial properties and might support respiratory health.
29. Oregano:- Function as a spicy kick. Oregano oil can have a strong, spicy aroma and might have antimicrobial properties.
30. Vetiver:- Like a calming forest stroll, Vetiver oil is grounding and has an earthy, woody scent that can promote relaxation.

The list goes on- these oils have their own unique scents and benefits, and people use them in various ways to improve well-being and create pleasant environments

Extraction Methods and Purity

Essential oils are extracted from plants through different methods. While doing things, expert says ensuring their purity is super important. These are the ways they can be extracted:

Distillation:- This is a common method where steam passes through the plant material, carrying the essential oil. When the steam cools, it separates into water and oil, and the oil is collected.

Expression or Cold Pressing:- This method is often used for citrus oils. It involves mechanically pressing the rinds of fruits to extract the oil.

Solvent Extraction:- Sometimes, solvents are used to get the oils out of plants. After extraction, the solvent is removed, leaving behind the essential oil.

The purity of every method used is key because it ensures that the oil only contains the good stuff from the plant without any added chemicals or contaminants. High-quality oils are usually pure and free from synthetic additives, ensuring they're safe and effective to use. To check for purity, look for oils that are labelled as **"100% pure"** and come from reputable sources that perform tests to guarantee quality.

What is Aromatherapy and its Benefits

Aromatherapy is like a spa day for your senses. It's a practice where essential oils, with their lovely scents, are used to help your mind and body feel awesome.

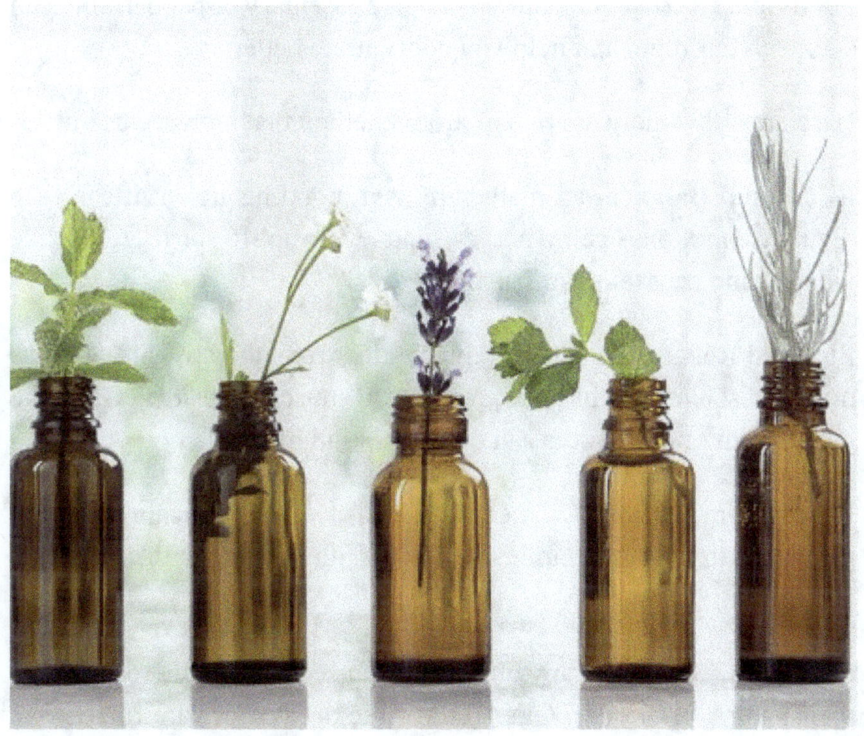

Here are some benefits gotten from the practice:

Relaxation:- Certain scents, like lavender or chamomile, can help you unwind after a long day and relax your mind.

Mood Boost:- Some oils, like citrus ones, can make you feel happier and more energized.

Stress Relief:- Aromatherapy can ease stress and tension. Oils like bergamot or frankincense can work wonders for this.

Better Sleep:- Lavender is a superstar here. It can help you drift off to dreamland and have a more restful sleep.

Focus and **Clarity**:- Certain scents, like rosemary or peppermint, can sharpen your mind and help you concentrate better.

Here are a few more aspects of aromatherapy that are very useful:-

Emotional Balance- aromatherapy is a mood magician, it can help regulate emotions, calm nerves, and even uplift spirits. Oils like ylang-ylang or jasmine are great for this.

Physical Relief- as a natural remedy kit, Aromatherapy oils can ease minor discomforts like headaches or muscle tension. Oils like peppermint or eucalyptus can offer this kind of relief.

Respiratory Support- Some oils, such as tea tree or eucalyptus, have properties that can support respiratory health, helping with congestion or breathing issues.

Skin Care- Aromatherapy oils are often used in skincare routines for their natural properties. Oils like tea tree or lavender are fingered in this area for their soothing and other benefits to the skin.

Holistic Healing- Aromatherapy is about treating the mind, body, and spirit. It's like a gentle, holistic approach to feeling better inside and out

Aromatherapy is versatile and can be enjoyed in many ways, like using diffusers, adding oils to baths, or even just inhaling the scent from a few drops on a tissue.

Knowledge Behind Essential Oils

The science behind essential oils is pretty cool. These oils are made up of tiny molecules that carry the unique scents and properties of plants. Here's the gist:

Chemical Composition:- Essential oils are made of various natural chemicals that give them their specific smell and effects. Each oil has its own special mix of these chemicals, like terpenes or phenols.

How They Work:- When you smell an essential oil, those tiny molecules go up your nose and can interact with the olfactory system. This interaction can affect your brain, and emotions, and even trigger memories. It's why certain scents can make you feel relaxed or happier.

Absorption:- When applied to the skin (usually diluted), these molecules can also be absorbed and get into your bloodstream. This is why some oils, like lavender or tea tree, are used in skincare- they can have beneficial effects.

Effects on the Body:- Some oils have properties that can help with things like inflammation, and pain, or even have antibacterial or antifungal effects.

Safety Precautions:- Because they're super concentrated, essential oils need to be used carefully. Too much of a strong oil can sometimes cause irritation or adverse reactions, so it's important to use them properly and in the right amounts.

Scientists are still learning more about essential oils and their effects on the body, but their natural properties and potential benefits are pretty fascinating.

How Essential Oils Work in the Body

Essential oils are pretty amazing when it comes to how they work in the human body. Or how we use them to derive the benefit they offer. this reminds me of the following:

Inhalation:- When you breathe in the scent of essential oils, they travel through your nose and can interact with your olfactory system. This interaction sends signals to your brain, affecting your emotions, mood, and even memory.

Absorption process:- When diluted oil is applied to the skin, some molecules from the essential oils can be absorbed. They can pass through the skin and enter your bloodstream. This is why certain oils, like lavender or peppermint, are used in massage or skincare.

Effect on **Cells**:- Once in the bloodstream, the molecules from essential oils can interact with cells and body systems. Some oils have properties that can help with inflammation, pain relief, or even support the immune system.

Emotional and **Mental Effects**:- Essential oils can have a powerful impact on emotions, help calm nerves, reduce stress, and boost mood—all through the interaction of scent with your brain.

Supporting Wellness:- Certain oils have properties that might support overall well-being. For example, tea tree oil is known for its antibacterial properties, while eucalyptus oil can help with congestion.

It's pretty incredible how these natural plant extracts can have effects on both the body and mind, offering potential benefits for various aspects of our health and wellness.

General Safety Precautions on How to Use Essential Oil

Safety is crucial when using essential oils. Here are some important precautions and usage guidelines in order to get the best from the oil:

Dilution:- Essential oils are highly concentrated, so it's vital to dilute them before applying them to the skin. Mix them with a carrier oil like coconut, almond, or jojoba oil. This helps prevent skin irritation or sensitivity reactions.

Patch Test:- Before using a new essential oil, do a patch test by applying a small diluted amount on a small area of skin and waiting to see if there's any adverse reaction over 24 hours.

Avoiding Sensitive Areas:- Keep oils away from sensitive areas like eyes, ears, or mucous membranes. If accidental contact occurs, flush the area with a carrier oil, **not water**, to dilute it.

Storage:- Proper Storage of essential oils is important, best stored in dark, glass bottles away from direct sunlight or heat. This helps preserve their potency.

Pregnancy and **Children**:- Some essential oils might not be safe during pregnancy or for young children. Always check with a healthcare professional before using oils in these situations.

Usage Amounts or **Dosages**:- Less is often more with essential oils. Use only a few drops in a diffuser or when blending them for topical application.

Quality Matters:- Ensure you're using high-quality, pure essential oils from reputable sources. Avoid synthetic fragrances or adulterated oils.

If you have any health conditions or are taking medications, it's a good idea to consult with a healthcare professional before using essential oils to avoid any potential interactions. Respecting these guidelines helps ensure that you can enjoy the benefits of essential oils safely and effectively.

Practical Application of Essential Oil

Essential oils have various practical applications that can be part of your daily routine which have already been mentioned in **Aromatherapy**, **Body Massage**, **Skincare**, **Bathing**, **Cleaning**, **Inhalation**, and **DIY Projects** like getting creative with essential oils-recall that it is used in homemade candles, soaps, or skincare products for personalized, natural alternative.

Some Ailments and Corresponding Oils

Here are some common ailments and the corresponding essential oils that are often used to help for relief:-

Headaches:- people use peppermint, Lavender, and Eucalyptus - Apply diluted peppermint oil on temples or use a cool compress. Lavender oil can be calming, and eucalyptus may help ease tension.

Stress and **Anxiety**:- Lavender, Chamomile, and Frankincense can be helpful. Use them in a diffuser, add to bathwater, or use in massage oils.

Congestion:- Eucalyptus, Peppermint, and Tea Tree come in handy. Inhale steam with a few drops of eucalyptus or peppermint oil. Tea tree oil may help with respiratory issues.

Muscle Pain:- Peppermint, Lavender, Rosemary - Mix with a carrier oil and massage onto sore muscles for relief.

Skin Irritations:- Tea Tree, Lavender, and Chamomile are useful for soothing minor skin issues. Dilute and apply to affected areas.

Sleep Troubles:- Lavender, Roman Chamomile, and Valerian will suffice. Use in a diffuser, apply diluted oil to pulse points, or add a few drops to a pillow for a calming sleep aid.

If you have sensitive skin or if you have allergies, apply cautiously. If symptoms persist or worsen, it's best to consult a healthcare professional.

Some Do It Yourself Remedies and Recipes

Here are some simple DIY remedies and recipes for lovers of essential oils:

Soothing Massage Oil:-

Ingredients:- 2-3 drops of lavender oil, 2-3 drops of chamomile oil, 1 oz (30ml) of carrier oil (like almond or jojoba oil).

Mix the essential oils with the carrier oil in a bottle. Use it for a relaxing massage.

Refreshing Room Spray:-

Ingredients:- 10-15 drops of lemon oil, 10-15 drops of peppermint oil, distilled water.

Add the essential oils to a spray bottle and fill it up with distilled water. Shake well before each use and spritz in your room for a fresh scent.

Relaxing Bath Salts:-

Ingredients:- 1 cup Epsom salts, 5-10 drops of lavender oil, 3-5 drops of cedarwood oil.

Mix the essential oils with Epsom salts in a bowl. Add to your bath for a calming soak.

Homemade Vapor Rub:-

Ingredients:- 1/4 cup coconut oil, 10 drops of eucalyptus oil, 5 drops of peppermint oil, 5 drops of rosemary oil.

Melt the coconut oil, add essential oils, mix, and store in a jar. Rub on the chest or throat for congestion relief.

All-Purpose Cleaning Spray:-

Ingredients:- 15-20 drops tea tree oil, 10-15 drops lemon oil, 1 cup distilled white vinegar, water.

Mix the oils with vinegar in a spray bottle and fill it up with water. Use it as an effective, natural cleaner for surfaces.

Always ensure to store DIY mixtures in dark glass bottles away from direct sunlight, and label them properly. Also, perform a patch test before using any new mixture on your skin to check for sensitivity or allergies.

Incorporating Essential Oils into Daily Life

Incorporating essential oils into your daily routine can be fun and beneficial. Here are some easy ways to do it:-

Diffusing:- Use an essential oil diffuser in your home or office. Add a few drops of your favourite oil or a blend to the diffuser for a lovely aroma.

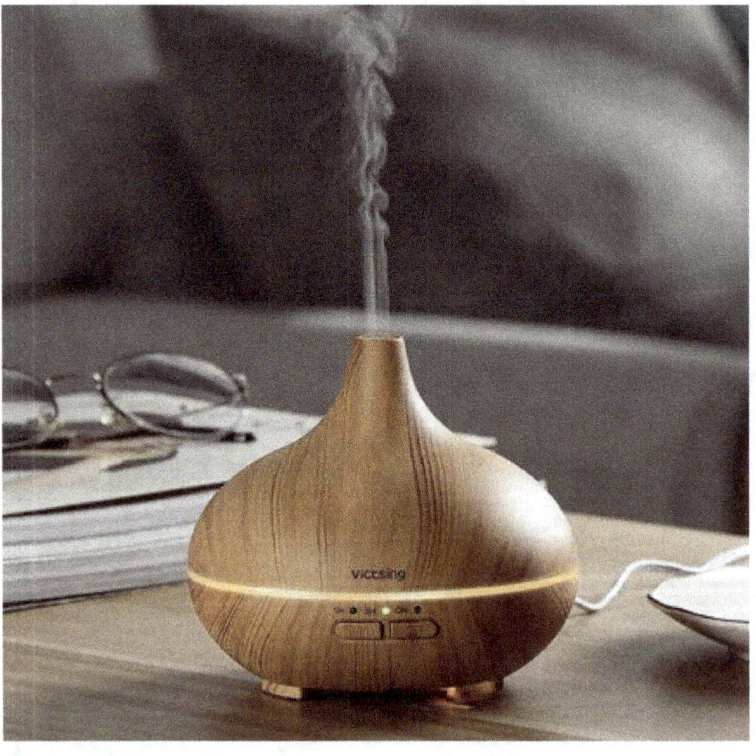

Morning Boost:- Add a drop of citrus oil (like lemon or orange) to your shower gel for a refreshing start to your day.

Desk De-stress:- Keep a small rollerball with diluted lavender or peppermint oil at your desk. Roll it on your wrists or temples for a quick stress reliever during the day.

Skincare Routine:- Mix a drop or two of tea tree or lavender oil into your facial cleanser or moisturizer for added benefits.

Bedtime Ritual:- Diffuse calming oils like lavender or chamomile before bedtime for a relaxing atmosphere. You can also add a drop of lavender oil to your pillow.

Laundry Boost:- Add a few drops of your preferred oil to wool dryer balls before starting your laundry for a natural, fresh scent.

Yoga or Meditation:- Use oils like frankincense or sandalwood during your yoga or meditation practice for a grounding effect.

DIY Air Freshener:- Create your own air freshener spray by mixing water and a few drops of essential oils in a spray bottle. Use it to freshen up rooms or linens.

Remember, start with small amounts and always dilute oils properly, especially when applying them to your skin. Experiment and find what works best for you.

Other Uses of Essential Oils at Home

Using essential oils at home can make your space smell amazing and bring numerous benefits:-

- Diffusers can disperse scents throughout your home. Add a few drops of your favourite oil or create your own blend for a pleasant aroma.

- Make homemade cleaning products by adding essential oils like tea tree, lemon, or eucalyptus to vinegar or water for a natural and fresh-smelling cleaner.
- Laundry- Add a few drops of essential oil to wool dryer balls or a damp cloth and toss them in the dryer to naturally freshen up the laundry.
- Linens and Fabrics- Spritz a mix of water and a few drops of essential oils on curtains, pillows, or bedding to infuse them with a pleasant scent.
- Candles- Add a few drops of essential oils to unscented candles before lighting them for a subtle fragrance.
- Drawer Sachets- Place cotton balls scented with essential oils in drawers or closets to keep clothes smelling fresh.
- Room Spray- Make a simple room spray by mixing water and essential oils in a spray bottle. Spritz it around to freshen up the air.

Cleaning and Purifying Spaces

Essential oils can be used effectively to clean and purify spaces naturally. Here's how:-

Surface Cleaning:- Create a natural cleaning spray by mixing water with essential oils known for their antibacterial properties, such as tea tree, lemon, or eucalyptus. Use this solution to clean countertops, tables, and other surfaces.

Air Purification:- Diffuse essential oils like tea tree, eucalyptus, or thyme to help cleanse the air of impurities, neutralize odours, and create a fresher environment.

Mould and Mildew Prevention:- Tea tree oil is especially effective against mould and mildew. Mix it with water in a spray bottle and apply to areas prone to mould growth, such as bathrooms or damp corners.

Natural Disinfectant:- Lemon oil, with its antimicrobial properties, can be added to homemade cleaning solutions. It not only leaves a fresh scent but also helps disinfect surfaces.

Deodorizing Carpets and Upholstery:- Sprinkle baking soda infused with a few drops of essential oils (like lavender or tea tree) on carpets or upholstery. Let it sit for a while before vacuuming to freshen and deodorize.

Trash Can Refresher:- Drop a few cotton balls with a few drops of essential oil at the bottom of your trash can to combat unpleasant odours.

Laundry Freshener:- Add a few drops of your favourite essential oil to a damp cloth and toss it in the dryer with your laundry for a natural fresh scent.

Essential Oils in Cooking and Recipes

Essential oils can add delightful flavours to your cooking. Here are some tips and ideas for using essential oils in recipes:-

Choose Wisely:- Not all essential oils are safe for consumption, so make sure you're using oils labelled as food-grade or suitable for culinary use.

Start Small:- Essential oils are highly concentrated, so start with just a drop or two. You can always add more, but you can't take it away once it's in the dish.

Dilution is Key:- Due to their potency, it's best to dilute essential oils before using them in cooking. You can mix them with carrier oil, honey, or other liquids.

Citrus Zest Replacement:- Essential oils from citrus fruits like lemon, orange, or lime can replace zest in recipes. One drop of oil usually equals about one teaspoon of zest.

Flavour Enhancers:- Oils like peppermint, basil, rosemary, or oregano can add a punch of flavour to dishes. For example, a drop of basil oil in tomato sauce or a drop of peppermint oil in chocolate recipes can be delightful.

Drinks and Beverages:- Add a drop of citrus oil to water, tea, or cocktails for a burst of flavour. For instance, a drop of lemon oil in a glass of water can be refreshing.

Infusions and Marinades:- Use essential oils to infuse oils, marinades, or salad dressings. A drop of rosemary oil in olive oil for a herb-infused flavour or a drop of ginger oil in a marinade can be wonderful.

Baking:- Add a drop of cinnamon, nutmeg, or other spice oils to baked goods for a flavorful twist.

Remember, a little goes a long way with essential oils in cooking. Experiment with caution and have fun exploring how these oils can elevate the flavours of your dishes.

Herbaceous Flavors:- Oils like basil, rosemary, thyme, oregano, and dill can bring robust herb flavours to savoury dishes, soups, sauces, and marinades.

Minty Freshness:- Peppermint and spearmint oils can add a refreshing twist to desserts, beverages, chocolates, and even savoury dishes like salads or sauces.

Spice Infusion:- Essential oils like cinnamon, ginger, nutmeg, clove, and cardamom can be used in baking, hot beverages, curries, and desserts for a warming, aromatic touch.

Tropical Sensations:- Coconut, pineapple, mango, and other tropical fruit oils can be used in smoothies, desserts, or marinades to impart tropical flavours.

Floral Notes:- Lavender, jasmine, and rose oils can delicately flavour desserts, teas, syrups, or even savoury dishes for a unique floral touch.

Savoury Blends:- Blends like Italian seasoning (a mix of basil, oregano, thyme, rosemary) or Herbs de Provence (thyme, rosemary, marjoram, lavender) can elevate the flavours of various dishes.

Safety and Proper Usage of Food

Even Distribution:- Since oils don't mix well with water, it's best to blend them with fats or oils first. Mixing them with butter, honey, or oils like olive or coconut before adding them to your recipe helps ensure even distribution.

Start Small:- When using essential oils in cooking, start with a minimal amount and gradually increase as needed. It's easier to add more, but difficult to reduce if you've added too much.

Know Your Oils:- Some essential oils are stronger than others, so be cautious with potent oils like cinnamon, clove, or peppermint. They can easily overpower a dish if used excessively.

Avoid Heating Excessively:- Essential oils can lose their potency or alter their flavour profile when exposed to high heat for extended periods. It's best to add them towards the end of cooking or use them in no-cook recipes.

Specific Uses:- Certain oils are more suited for specific types of dishes. For instance, citrus oils work well in desserts and beverages, while herb oils are great in savoury dishes.

Allergies and Sensitivities:- Be mindful of any allergies or sensitivities to specific oils. When serving dishes with essential oils, inform guests about their presence.

Chapter 4

Essential Oils for Different Lifestyles

Athletes and Fitness Enthusiasts

Essential oils can be beneficial for athletes and fitness enthusiasts in various ways:-

Pre-Workout Energizer:- Citrus oils like lemon or orange can provide a natural energy boost. Inhaling or diffusing these oils before a workout may help improve focus and motivation.

Muscle Relief:- Oils such as peppermint, eucalyptus, or wintergreen, when diluted with a carrier oil, can be massaged onto muscles post-workout to soothe soreness and provide a cooling sensation.

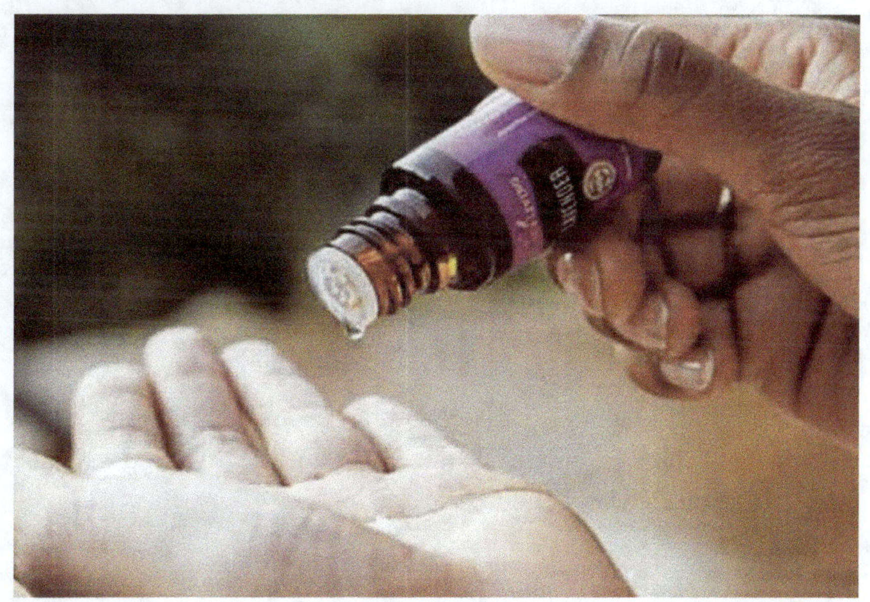

Respiratory Support:- Eucalyptus or tea tree oils, when diffused, can help clear the airways, making breathing easier during workouts, especially for cardio exercises.

Mental Focus:- Essential oils like rosemary or peppermint may help enhance mental clarity and concentration. Diffuse them or use them as a personal inhaler before workouts to improve focus.

Stress Relief:- Lavender, chamomile, or frankincense oils can aid in relaxation. After intense workouts, diffusing these oils may help in calming down and promoting better sleep.

DIY Workout Gear:- Add a few drops of essential oils to homemade workout gear cleaners or yoga mat sprays for a fresh and clean-smelling exercise environment.

Recovery Baths:- Adding a few drops of lavender or chamomile oil to a post-workout bath can help relax muscles and ease tension.

Families and Children

Essential oils can be beneficial for families and children, but extra caution is needed when using them around young ones:-

Supporting Immunity:- Tea tree, eucalyptus, or frankincense oils have properties that might support the immune system. They can be diffused to cleanse the air during cold and flu seasons.

DIY Natural Cleaners:- Create natural cleaning solutions using essential oils like tea tree or lemon. They're effective and safe for cleaning surfaces where children play.

Consultation with Healthcare Providers:- If children have underlying health conditions or allergies, or if you're pregnant or nursing, consult a healthcare provider before using essential oils.

Keep essential oils out of reach of children and ensure proper storage. Always follow safety guidelines and use oils cautiously around infants and young children.

Seniors and Elderly Care

Essential oils can offer benefits for seniors and elderly care, but it's crucial to use them with caution too, especially considering any existing health conditions or medications. Here are some considerations:-

Aromatherapy for Relaxation:- Lavender, chamomile, or geranium oils that promote relaxation may help seniors unwind or manage stress.

Joint and Muscle Support:- Oils like peppermint, eucalyptus, or ginger can provide relief for sore muscles or joint discomfort when diluted and applied topically.

Respiratory Support:- Eucalyptus, tea tree, or lemon oils can be diffused to support respiratory health and ease breathing for seniors dealing with congestion or respiratory issues.

Sleep Aid:- Lavender and cedarwood oils may promote better sleep quality. Diffusing these oils in the bedroom can create a calming environment for a more restful sleep.

Cautious Application:- Dilute oils heavily and perform patch tests on a small area of skin before applying to ensure no adverse reactions, especially as skin sensitivity might increase with age.

Consult Healthcare Providers if seniors have medical conditions, are taking medications, or have allergies, before using essential oils.

Use minimal amounts and low-intensity diffusion to avoid overwhelming scents, which could potentially cause discomfort for seniors with heightened sensitivities.

Avoid accidental ingestion, when used cautiously and with proper guidance, essential oils can offer a natural and soothing support to the well-being of seniors.

Blending Essential Oils for Specific Purposes

Blending essential oils can create synergistic effects, enhancing their individual properties. Here are some blends for specific purposes:-

Relaxation Blend:-

- Lavender:- 3 drops
- Chamomile:- 2 drops
- Cedarwood:- 2 drops

Dilute in a carrier oil for a calming massage blend or use in a diffuser before bedtime.

Energizing Blend:-

- Peppermint:- 2 drops
- Orange:- 3 drops

- Rosemary:- 2 drops

Diffuse this blend to create a refreshing and energizing atmosphere.

Focus and Concentration Blend:-

- Lemon:- 3 drops
- Frankincense:- 2 drops
- Basil:- 2 drops

Diffuse during work or study sessions for enhanced focus.

Respiratory Support Blend:-

- Eucalyptus:- 3 drops
- Tea Tree:- 2 drops
- Lemon:- 2 drops

Use a diffuser to help clear the airways during times of congestion.

Muscle Relief Blend:-

- Peppermint:- 3 drops
- Lavender:- 2 drops
- Marjoram:- 2 drops

Dilute in a carrier oil and massage onto sore muscles.

Mood Uplifting Blend:-

- Bergamot:- 3 drops
- Ylang Ylang:- 2 drops
- Geranium:- 2 drops

Diffuse this blend for a cheerful and uplifting atmosphere.

Exploring Unconventional Uses

Essential oils have unconventional uses beyond aromatherapy or skincare. Here are some unique ways to explore their versatility:-

DIY Bug Repellent:- Certain oils like citronella, lemongrass, or tea tree can be used in homemade bug sprays to repel insects when diluted with water or a carrier oil.

Removing Sticky Residue:- Apply a small amount of lemon oil to remove sticky residue from surfaces like glass, labels, or adhesives.

Freshening Shoes:- Place a few drops of tea tree oil on cotton balls and tuck them into shoes to help eliminate odour and keep them smelling fresh.

Enhancing Laundry:- Add a drop of lavender or lemon oil to a damp cloth and toss it into the dryer with laundry for a natural fresh scent.

Reviving Potpourri:- Add a few drops of essential oils to dried potpourri to refresh its scent and revive its potency.

Enhancing Wooden Furniture:- Mix lemon or orange oil with carrier oil to polish and protect wooden furniture naturally.

Refreshing Trash Cans:- Put a few drops of pine, eucalyptus, or tea tree oil on a cotton ball and place it at the bottom of the trash can to neutralize odours.

Creating Natural Reed Diffusers:- Combine essential oils with a carrier oil and place the mixture in a bottle with reed sticks for a DIY air freshener.

Scenting Stationery:- Apply a drop of essential oil to a cotton ball and tuck it into a drawer with stationery or books for a pleasant fragrance.

Enhancing Bathwater:- Mix a few drops of essential oils with a carrier oil or Epsom salts before adding to bathwater for a spa-like experience.

Chapter 5

My Exploration with Essential Oil Extraction Methods

I've delved into various methods for extracting essential oils in the past, and while some traditional methods are still widely used, they have their drawbacks. Conventional techniques often pose challenges like the degradation of certain compounds and the loss of components. It's however promising to hear about ongoing efforts to refine these methods, selecting them based on the plant and desired product quality.

Each extraction technique as discussed here offers distinct advantages and limitations, influencing the composition of essential oils and the overall yield. Let me walk you through some of these methods and their intricacies.

Steam Extraction

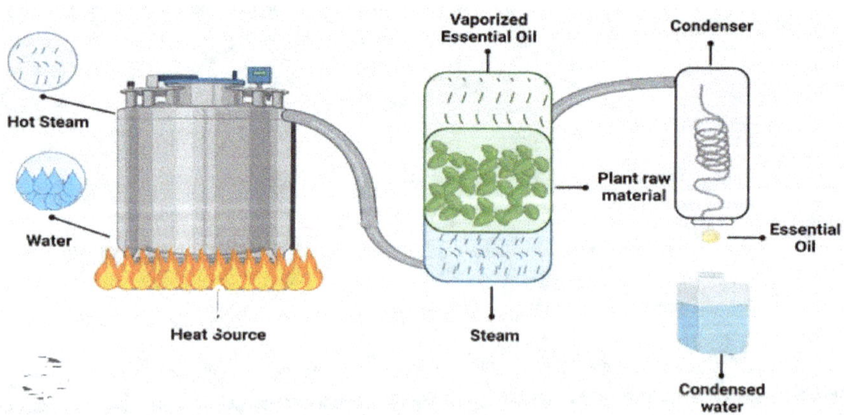

For instance, steam extraction is a widely accepted method that uses steam to release essential oils from plant material. This process, lasting from 1 to 10 hours, depends on factors such as time, temperature, and pressure, retrieving about 95% of the volatile molecules within half an hour.

Hydrodistillation

On the other hand, hydrodistillation involves immersing plant material in water and boiling it. Though effective, it can lead to overheating, especially for delicate floral materials, resulting in burned-smelling oils.

Hydrodiffusion

Hydrodiffusion is a gentler approach that uses steam and water, particularly suited for delicate plant materials. It operates at lower temperatures and less pressure compared to other methods.

Cold Pressing and Enfleurage

Cold pressing is a classic method for extracting citrus peel oils, while enfleurage, though ancient, remains an option for flowers with long-lasting fragrances.

Organic Solvent Extraction

Solvent extraction, while efficient, involves the use of solvents like hexane or acetone. It's fast but comes with risks due to solvent residue in the final product.

Newer "Green" Techniques

Recent advancements in extraction include microwave-assisted methods, like microwave solvent-assisted extraction. This innovative technique reduces extraction times and solvent consumption, making it more environmentally friendly.

Supercritical Fluid Extraction

Supercritical fluid extraction (SFE) is another cutting-edge approach that uses substances above their critical temperature and pressure as solvents. This method yields higher selectivity and reduced solvent use, but careful pressure management is crucial to avoid extracting unwanted compounds.

Each of these techniques has its place in the world of essential oil extraction, offering unique benefits and challenges. The newer "green" methods, especially, show promising strides towards more sustainable and efficient extraction practices.

There's quite a variety of these extraction methods, each with its own strengths and considerations. If you want to go deeper into any particular method, just consult relevant professionals and learn more about the process.

such as moisture, warmth, and nutrients. Moreover, the sprouting process itself can sometimes compromise the natural defenses of the seed against pathogens....

Seed Contamination...

Contaminated seeds are a primary source of sprout-related outbreaks. Even when seeds are tested and sanitized, there can be residual pathogens. Additionally, seeds can become contaminated during the growth process or through contact with contaminated water or equipment....

Commercial vs. Home Sprouting...

While commercial sprout producers follow strict guidelines to minimize contamination risks, home sprouting carries higher risks due to potentially less stringent sanitation practices. Those who choose to sprout at home should be aware of the importance of using high-quality seeds and following recommended safety practices....

Regulatory Measures...

Regulatory bodies like the FDA and EFSA have implemented measures to address sprout safety. These measures include seed testing, sanitation practices, and monitoring of sprout production facilities. Despite these efforts, outbreaks still occur, highlighting the challenges associated with ensuring the safety of sprouts....

Conclusion...

Chapter 4 has provided an in-depth look at the contaminants and pathogens that have been responsible for sprout-related foodborne illnesses. While sprouts offer numerous health benefits, it's essential to be aware of the potential risks and the importance of safe sprouting practices. In the following chapters, we will explore strategies for growing sprouts safely at home and the regulatory measures in place to mitigate risks. Join us in Chapter 5 as we delve into the practical aspects of growing sprouts in a home setting....

Chapter 5: Growing Sprouts Safely at Home...

For those who are enthusiastic about the nutritional benefits of sprouts and want to enjoy them at home, this chapter provides valuable insights into growing sprouts safely. By following recommended practices, you can minimize the risks associated with home sprouting....

Selecting High-Quality Seeds...

The foundation of safe sprouting at home begins with the seeds themselves. It's essential to choose high-quality seeds from reputable suppliers. Look for seeds labeled as specifically intended for sprouting, as they are subject to quality controls and testing for contaminants....

Equipment and Supplies...

To start home sprouting, you'll need minimal equipment and supplies, including:...

Glass jars or sprouting trays: These provide a suitable environment for sprouting....

Seeds: As mentioned, ensure they are high-quality sprouting seeds....

Water: Use clean, filtered water....

A fine mesh strainer: To rinse and drain sprouts....

Clean cloth or paper towels: For covering and shading sprouts during germination....

Hygiene and Sanitation...

Maintaining cleanliness during the sprouting process is crucial. Here are some key hygiene and sanitation practices to follow:...

Wash hands: Always wash your hands thoroughly before handling seeds or sprouts....

Sanitize equipment: Ensure that jars, trays, and utensils are clean and sanitized before use....

Rinse seeds: Rinse seeds well before sprouting to remove any residual contaminants....

Sprouting Methods...

There are various methods for sprouting at home, including jar sprouting, tray sprouting, and even sprouting bags. Choose the method that suits your preferences and available equipment....

Proper Rinsing and Draining...

During the sprouting process, it's crucial to rinse and drain the sprouts regularly, typically two to three times a day. This helps prevent the growth of harmful microorganisms by removing excess moisture....

Monitoring Temperature and Humidity...

Maintain appropriate temperature and humidity levels for sprouting. Most sprouts thrive in room temperature conditions, away from direct sunlight. Keeping sprouting containers in a well-ventilated area is also essential....

Harvesting and Storage...

Harvest sprouts when they have reached the desired length, typically around 1-2 inches. Rinse them one final time and allow them to drain thoroughly. Store sprouts in the refrigerator to maintain freshness....

Safe Sprout Consumption...

Before enjoying your homegrown sprouts, it's a good practice to give them a final rinse. You can add sprouts to salads, sandwiches, wraps, or even use them as a garnish for various dishes....

Conclusion...

Growing sprouts safely at home is entirely achievable with the right seeds, equipment, and adherence to hygiene practices. While there are inherent risks associated with sprouting, following these guidelines can significantly reduce those risks. In the following chapters, we will explore regulatory measures and guidelines designed to enhance the safety of commercially produced sprouts. Join us in Chapter 6 as we examine the regulations and standards in place to safeguard sprout production....

Chapter 6: Regulatory Measures and Guidelines...

The safety of commercially produced sprouts relies on a combination of regulatory measures and industry guidelines. In this chapter, we'll explore the various standards and regulations in place to ensure the safety of sprouts available in the market....

The Role of Regulatory Bodies...

Regulatory bodies, such as the U.S. Food and Drug Administration (FDA) and the European Food Safety Authority (EFSA), play a crucial role in overseeing the safety of sprouts and other food products. Their responsibilities include:...

Inspection and Monitoring...

Regulatory agencies conduct routine inspections of sprout production facilities to assess compliance with safety standards. They may also sample and test sprouts for contaminants....

Setting Safety Standards...

Regulatory bodies establish and update safety standards for sprout production. These standards cover various aspects, including seed quality, sanitation, and monitoring of production facilities....

Recall Management...

In the event of a suspected or confirmed contamination, regulatory agencies work with sprout producers to initiate recalls and remove unsafe products from the market....

Key Regulatory Measures...

Seed Testing...

One critical aspect of sprout safety is seed testing. Regulatory guidelines often require sprout producers to use seeds that have undergone pathogen testing to ensure they are free from harmful microorganisms....

Sanitation Practices...

Commercial sprout production facilities must adhere to stringent sanitation practices. This includes maintaining clean and hygienic production environments, regularly cleaning equipment, and ensuring water quality....

Water Treatment...

Water used in sprout production must meet specific quality standards. Many outbreaks have been linked to contaminated water sources, highlighting the importance of treating water used for irrigation and rinsing....

Temperature Control...

Controlling temperature is crucial during sprout production. Maintaining the right temperature conditions can inhibit the growth of pathogens and reduce the risk of contamination....

Industry Guidelines...

In addition to regulatory measures, industry organizations often develop guidelines to enhance the safety of sprouts. These guidelines may include best practices for sprout production, handling, and transportation....

Challenges and Ongoing Concerns...

Despite the efforts of regulatory bodies and industry organizations, challenges related to sprout safety persist. Contaminated seeds, water quality issues, and the unique growth conditions of sprouts continue to pose risks....

Conclusion...

Chapter 6 has shed light on the regulatory measures and guidelines that govern the safety of commercially produced sprouts. While these measures aim to minimize risks, it's essential for consumers to remain informed about sprout safety and to follow recommended practices when purchasing and handling sprouts. In the chapters ahead, we will further explore the science behind sprout safety and examine common myths and misconceptions. Join us in Chapter 7 as we delve into the scientific principles that underpin sprout safety....

Chapter 7: The Science Behind Sprout Safety...

To truly understand sprout safety, it's essential to explore the scientific principles that underlie the potential risks and mitigating factors. In this chapter, we will delve into the biology and microbiology of sprouts to gain insights into the factors influencing their safety....

The Sprouting Process...

Sprouting is a complex biological process that transforms seeds into young plants. During sprouting, the dormant seed awakens, and various biochemical changes occur:...

Germination: The process begins with soaking the seeds in water, triggering the seed to absorb water and initiate growth....

Enzymatic Activity: As the seed begins to sprout, enzymes are activated. These enzymes break down complex nutrients within the seed into simpler forms that the developing plant can use for growth....

Growth and Nutrient Accumulation: The young plant develops, and its nutrient content increases as it absorbs minerals and vitamins from the seed....

Ideal Conditions for Growth...

Sprouts thrive in warm and humid conditions, which are also favorable for the growth of microorganisms, including potential pathogens. The moist environment created during sprouting can become a breeding ground for bacteria if proper precautions are not taken....

Microbial Concerns...

Microorganisms, such as Salmonella, E. coli, and Listeria, are the primary concerns when it comes to sprout safety. Here's how these microorganisms can enter and grow within sprouts:...

Seed Contamination:
Microorganisms may reside on the

surface of seeds, and if not adequately disinfected, they can multiply during the sprouting process....

Water: Contaminated water used for irrigation or rinsing can introduce pathogens to the sprouts....

Sprouting Environment: The warm, humid conditions during sprouting are ideal for bacterial growth. If pathogens are present, they can multiply rapidly....

Preventing Microbial Growth...

Effective prevention of microbial growth in sprouts involves:...

Seed Sanitation: Thorough cleaning and, in some cases,

disinfection of seeds before sprouting....

Water Quality: Ensuring that water used in sprouting is of high quality and free from contaminants....

Temperature Control: Maintaining appropriate temperature conditions to inhibit bacterial growth....

Hygiene: Strict adherence to hygiene practices by sprout producers and handlers....

Conclusion...

Chapter 7 has provided an insight into the science behind sprout safety, including the biological processes of sprouting and the microbial concerns associated with this unique food. As we continue our journey through this book, we will address common myths and misconceptions surrounding sprouts. Join us in Chapter 8 as we debunk some of the misconceptions and present evidence-based information about sprouts....

Chapter 8: Common Myths and Misconceptions...

The world of sprouts is not immune to myths and misconceptions. In this chapter, we will separate fact from fiction by addressing and debunking some of the common misconceptions surrounding sprouts....

Myth 1: All Sprouts Are Unsafe to Eat...

Fact: While there have been concerns about the safety of sprouts due to past outbreaks, not all sprouts are inherently unsafe. The safety of sprouts depends on various factors, including seed quality, production practices, and hygiene. When produced and handled correctly, sprouts can be safe to consume....

Myth 2: Cooking Sprouts Eliminates All Risks...

Fact: Cooking sprouts can significantly reduce the risk of foodborne illness by killing most harmful microorganisms. However, it's important to start with clean and safe sprouts. Cooking contaminated sprouts may not guarantee safety, as some pathogens can be heat-resistant....

Myth 3: Sprouts Lack Nutritional Value...

Fact: Quite the contrary! Sprouts are packed with essential nutrients, including vitamins, minerals, and antioxidants. They are a valuable addition to a balanced diet and offer numerous health benefits when properly prepared and consumed....

Myth 4: Homegrown Sprouts Are Always Safe...

Fact: While growing sprouts at home can be safe when proper practices are followed, there are inherent risks. Contaminated seeds, poor hygiene, and improper sprouting conditions can still lead to foodborne illness. Home sprouters should be aware of these risks and take necessary precautions....

Myth 5: Sprouts Are Only for Salads...

Fact: Sprouts are incredibly versatile and can be used in various dishes beyond salads. They add crunch, flavor, and nutrition to sandwiches, wraps, stir-fries, soups, and more. Get creative and experiment with different culinary applications....

Myth 6: Sprouts Are Always a Source of Foodborne Illness...

Fact: While sprouts have been associated with foodborne illness outbreaks, it's essential to recognize that many food products, including meat and seafood, can also pose food safety risks. Awareness of best practices and proper handling can mitigate these risks....

Myth 7: Sprouts Are Not Suitable for Vulnerable Populations...

Fact: Vulnerable populations, such as pregnant women, can safely enjoy sprouts when they are cooked thoroughly. Cooking sprouts reduces the risk of foodborne illness and allows these individuals to benefit from the nutrients sprouts offer....

Conclusion...

In Chapter 8, we've debunked some common myths and misconceptions surrounding sprouts. Understanding the facts about sprouts and their safety is essential for making informed dietary choices. As we progress through this book, we will continue to explore various aspects of sprouts, including their cultivation, nutritional value, and practical applications. Join us in Chapter 9 as we discuss the science and techniques of growing sprouts at home....

Chapter 9: Growing Sprouts at Home - Techniques and Tips...

Now that we've explored the science, safety, and debunked myths surrounding sprouts, it's time to get hands-on with growing sprouts at home. In this chapter, we'll delve into the techniques, tips, and best practices for successfully cultivating sprouts in your own kitchen....

Selecting the Right Seeds...

The foundation of successful home sprouting begins with choosing the right seeds. Here's what you need to consider:...

Seed Quality: Opt for high-quality sprouting seeds that are specifically intended for sprouting. These seeds undergo testing and sanitation to reduce the risk of contamination....

Variety: There are various types of sprouting seeds, each with its own flavor and nutritional profile. Experiment with different varieties to find your favorites....

Equipment and Supplies...

You don't need an elaborate setup to sprout at home. Here are the basic items you'll need:...

Glass Jars or Sprouting Trays: These provide suitable environments for sprouting....

Seeds: Choose the seeds of your choice....

Clean Water: Use filtered or purified water for rinsing and soaking....

Fine Mesh Strainer: For rinsing and draining sprouts....

Clean Cloth or Paper Towels: To cover and shade sprouts during germination....

The Sprouting Process...

Here's a step-by-step guide to sprouting at home:...

Soaking: Start by soaking the seeds in clean water for the recommended time (usually 6-12 hours or as specified on the seed package). Soaking helps kickstart the germination process....

Rinsing: After soaking, rinse the seeds thoroughly under running water to remove any residue. Drain well....

Sprouting: Transfer the seeds to a glass jar or sprouting tray. Cover the container with a clean cloth or paper towel and secure it with a rubber band or string. This provides shade and prevents contamination....

Rinsing and Draining: Twice a day, rinse the sprouts with clean water and drain them thoroughly. This helps remove excess moisture and prevents bacterial growth....

Germination: Continue the rinsing and draining process until the sprouts have reached your desired length, typically 2-7 days, depending on the type of seed and desired sprout length....

Harvesting: Once your sprouts are ready, give them a final rinse and allow them to drain well. Harvest and enjoy!...

Tips for Success...

Maintain Hygiene: Ensure that your hands, equipment, and containers are clean and sanitized throughout the sprouting process....

Control Temperature: Keep sprouting containers in a well-ventilated area at room temperature, away from direct sunlight....

Experiment: Don't be afraid to experiment with different types of seeds and sprouting methods to find what works best for you....

Conclusion...

With the right seeds, equipment, and proper techniques, growing sprouts at home can be a rewarding and nutritious addition to your diet. In Chapter 10, we'll shift our focus to regulatory measures and guidelines for commercial sprout production. Understanding these standards will provide you with insights into the safety of store-bought sprouts....

Chapter 10: Regulatory Measures for Commercial Sprout Production...

As we continue our journey through the world of sprouts, this chapter focuses on the regulatory measures and guidelines that govern the safety of commercially produced sprouts. Understanding these standards is essential for consumers who purchase sprouts from stores or restaurants....

Regulatory Oversight...

Government agencies, such as the U.S. Food and Drug Administration (FDA) in the United States and the European Food Safety Authority (EFSA) in Europe, play a pivotal role in regulating the safety of commercial sprout production. Their responsibilities include:...

Inspection and Monitoring...

Regulatory bodies routinely inspect sprout production facilities to ensure compliance with safety standards. They may also conduct random testing of sprout samples for contaminants....

Setting Safety Standards...

Regulatory agencies establish and update safety standards for sprout production. These standards encompass various aspects, including seed quality, sanitation, and monitoring of production facilities....

Recalls and Enforcement...

In cases of confirmed contamination or safety violations, regulatory bodies work with sprout producers to initiate recalls, removing unsafe products from the market. Enforcement actions, such as fines and product seizures, may also be taken when necessary....

Key Regulatory Measures...

Seed Testing...

A fundamental aspect of sprout safety is seed testing. Regulatory guidelines often require sprout producers to use seeds that have undergone pathogen testing to ensure they are free from harmful microorganisms....

Sanitation Practices...

Commercial sprout production facilities must adhere to stringent sanitation practices. This includes maintaining clean and hygienic production environments, regular equipment cleaning, and ensuring water quality....

Water Treatment...

Water used in sprout production must meet specific quality

standards. Given that water is crucial for sprouting, ensuring its safety is paramount. Water treatment methods may include filtration and disinfection....

Temperature Control...

Maintaining appropriate temperature conditions is essential to inhibit bacterial growth during sprout production. This control helps minimize the risk of contamination....

Industry Guidelines...

In addition to regulatory measures, industry organizations often develop guidelines and best practices to further enhance the safety of sprout production. These guidelines may cover seed sourcing, testing, and production practices....

Challenges and Ongoing Concerns...

Despite regulatory efforts, challenges related to sprout safety continue. Contaminated seeds, water quality issues, and the unique growth conditions of sprouts can still pose risks. Consumer education remains a critical component of sprout safety....

Conclusion...

Chapter 10 has provided an overview of the regulatory measures and guidelines that govern the safety of commercially produced sprouts. When purchasing sprouts from stores or restaurants, consumers can have confidence that these products are subject to rigorous safety standards. In the chapters ahead, we will continue our exploration of sprouts, examining the future of sprout consumption and sharing personal stories and experiences related to this unique food. Join us in Chapter 11 as we discuss the evolving landscape of sprout consumption....

Chapter 11: The Future of Sprout Consumption...

As we move forward in our exploration of sprouts, it's crucial to consider the evolving landscape of sprout consumption. In this chapter, we'll delve into the future trends and innovations that may shape the way we view and enjoy sprouts in the years to come....

Growing Interest in Health and Sustainability...

Consumer awareness of health and sustainability is on the rise, and sprouts align with these trends perfectly:...

Nutritional Awareness: As people seek healthier dietary options, sprouts are gaining recognition for their nutrient-dense profiles. They are seen as a natural source of vitamins, minerals, and antioxidants....

Sustainable Farming: Sprouts are a sustainable food source, requiring fewer resources like water and land compared to fully grown vegetables. As environmental concerns grow, sprouts may become even more appealing....

Culinary Creativity...

Sprouts are versatile ingredients that can add texture, flavor, and nutrition to various dishes. Chefs and home cooks are experimenting with innovative ways to incorporate sprouts into their culinary creations:...

Fusion Cuisine: Sprouts are finding their way into fusion dishes that blend different culinary traditions, offering exciting flavor combinations....

Gourmet Offerings: High-end restaurants are featuring sprouts as

gourmet ingredients, elevating
their status beyond simple
garnishes....

DIY Food Movement...

The Do-It-Yourself (DIY) food
movement encourages people to
grow their own food, fostering a
deeper connection to what they
consume. Sprouting fits perfectly
within this movement:...

Home Gardening: Growing
sprouts at home allows individuals
to have control over the quality
and safety of their food....

Urban Farming: Sprouts are well-
suited for urban farming
initiatives, enabling city dwellers
to engage in small-scale
agriculture....

Food Safety Advancements...

As technology advances, so does our ability to enhance food safety:...

Seed Testing Innovations: Improved seed testing methods may reduce the risk of seed-related contamination....

Microbiome Research: A better understanding of the human microbiome may lead to personalized recommendations regarding sprout consumption for different individuals....

Conclusion...

The future of sprout consumption appears promising, with a growing emphasis on health, sustainability, culinary creativity, and DIY food production. As we continue our journey through this book, we will explore personal stories and experiences related to sprouts and share recipes featuring these nutritious greens. Join us in Chapter 12 as we dive into the personal narratives that shed light on the role of sprouts in individuals' lives....

Chapter 12: Personal Stories and Experiences with Sprouts...

Sprouts hold a special place in many people's lives, often associated with personal stories and memorable experiences. In this chapter, we'll delve into the narratives and accounts that shed light on the unique role sprouts play in individuals' lives....

A Journey to Better Health...

Sarah's Story:...

Sarah, a health-conscious individual, discovered sprouts while searching for nutrient-packed foods. She started incorporating sprouts into her daily diet, and over time, she noticed improvements in her overall health and vitality. Sprouts became a symbol of her journey to better well-being....

From Seed to Table...

David's Experience:...

David, an avid gardener, took his passion to the next level by growing sprouts at home. He found joy in nurturing seeds through the sprouting process and then savoring the fresh, homegrown sprouts on his plate. For David, sprouts represent the connection between the soil and the table....

Sprouts and Sustainability...

Ella's Perspective:...

Ella, an environmental advocate, appreciates sprouts not only for their nutritional value but also for their sustainability. She believes that choosing sprouts over resource-intensive vegetables is a small but meaningful step toward a more sustainable food system....

Culinary Adventures...

Carlos's Culinary Journey:...

Carlos, a chef with a passion for experimenting with ingredients, sees sprouts as a canvas for culinary creativity. He has crafted unique dishes that showcase the crunch and flavor of sprouts, delighting his customers and expanding their culinary horizons....

Sprouts in Cultural Traditions...

Lina's Cultural Connection:...

Lina, proud of her cultural heritage, incorporates sprouts into traditional dishes passed down through generations. For her, sprouts represent a bridge between her cultural roots and modern culinary practices....

Conclusion...

Personal stories and experiences with sprouts reveal the diverse ways in which this simple food can hold deep significance in people's lives. Whether it's a journey to better health, a connection to sustainability, a culinary adventure, or a cultural tie, sprouts continue to touch the lives of individuals in unique and meaningful ways....

In Chapter 13, we will explore practical tips and recipes to inspire your own sprout-based culinary adventures, encouraging you to embrace the versatility and nutritional benefits of sprouts in your everyday meals....

Chapter 13: Sprout-Based Culinary Adventures...

In this chapter, we embark on a culinary journey where sprouts take center stage. We'll explore practical tips and provide you with exciting recipes that showcase the versatility and nutritional benefits of sprouts in your everyday meals....

Tips for Preparing and Using Sprouts...

Before we dive into the recipes, here are some handy tips for preparing and using sprouts in your culinary creations:...

Rinse Thoroughly: Always rinse sprouts thoroughly before use to remove any residual contaminants and to freshen their flavor....

Trim as Needed: Trim the roots or any discolored portions of the sprouts, but be mindful not to remove too much, as that's where many of the nutrients are concentrated....

Mix and Match: Experiment with different types of sprouts to add variety to your dishes. Combining sprouts like alfalfa, broccoli, and radish can create a delightful mix of flavors and textures....

Texture Contrast: Use sprouts to add crunch and freshness to dishes that might otherwise lack textural contrast....

Add at the End: For cooked dishes, consider adding sprouts towards the end of the cooking process to retain their crispiness and nutritional value....

Recipe 1: Sprout and Avocado Salad...

Ingredients:...

cup mixed sprouts (alfalfa, broccoli, radish)...

ripe avocado, diced...

cup cherry tomatoes, halved...

1/4 cup red onion, finely chopped...

tablespoons lemon juice...

tablespoons olive oil...

Salt and pepper to taste...

Instructions:...

In a large bowl, combine the mixed sprouts, diced avocado, cherry tomatoes, and red onion....

In a separate small bowl, whisk together the lemon juice, olive oil, salt, and pepper to make the dressing....

Drizzle the dressing over the salad and gently toss to combine....

Serve immediately as a refreshing and nutritious salad....

Recipe 2: Sprout and Hummus Wrap...

Ingredients:...

4 large whole-grain tortillas...

cup hummus...

cups mixed sprouts (alfalfa, broccoli, radish)...

cucumber, thinly sliced...

red bell pepper, thinly sliced...

1/2 cup shredded carrots...

Salt and pepper to taste...

Instructions:...

Lay out the whole-grain tortillas on a clean surface....

Spread a generous layer of hummus onto each tortilla....

Arrange the mixed sprouts, cucumber slices, red bell pepper slices, and shredded carrots evenly over the hummus....

Season with salt and pepper to taste....

Roll up the tortillas tightly, securing the contents, and slice them in half....

These sprout and hummus wraps make a delicious and satisfying meal or snack....

Recipe 3: Stir-Fried Sprout Medley...

Ingredients:...

cups mixed sprouts (alfalfa, broccoli, radish)...

cup snap peas, trimmed...

cup sliced mushrooms...

red bell pepper, thinly sliced...

cloves garlic, minced...

tablespoons soy sauce...

tablespoon sesame oil...

teaspoon honey...

tablespoon sesame seeds (optional)...

Cooked rice or noodles for serving...

Instructions:...

In a small bowl, whisk together the soy sauce, sesame oil, and honey to create the stir-fry sauce....

Heat a large skillet or wok over medium-high heat. Add a splash of oil and sauté the minced garlic until fragrant....

Add the snap peas, mushrooms, and red bell pepper to the skillet. Stir-fry for a few minutes until they begin to soften....

Add the mixed sprouts to the skillet and continue to stir-fry for another 2-3 minutes until the sprouts are crisp-tender....

Pour the stir-fry sauce over the vegetables and toss to coat....

Serve the stir-fried sprout medley over cooked rice or noodles, and sprinkle with sesame seeds for added crunch and flavor....

Conclusion...

These recipes offer a taste of the culinary possibilities that sprouts bring to your kitchen. Whether in a refreshing salad, a hearty wrap, or a flavorful stir-fry, sprouts can elevate your meals with their nutritional value and unique texture. As we proceed to Chapter

14, we'll wrap up our exploration of sprouts by summarizing key takeaways and the enduring appeal of this versatile food....

Chapter 14: The Enduring Appeal of Sprouts...

In our final chapter, we reflect on the enduring appeal of sprouts and summarize the key takeaways from our journey through the world of sprouts. From their nutritional value to their role in culinary creativity, sprouts continue to capture our attention and offer a wealth of benefits....

Key Takeaways...

As we conclude our exploration of sprouts, let's recap some essential points:...

Nutritional Powerhouses: Sprouts are rich in vitamins, minerals, and antioxidants, making them a valuable addition to a healthy diet....

Safety First: While sprouts offer numerous health benefits, it's crucial to be aware of potential food safety risks associated with contamination....

Home Sprouting: Growing sprouts at home can be a rewarding and safe experience when following proper techniques and hygiene practices....

Regulatory Measures: Commercially produced sprouts are subject to rigorous safety standards and regulations to ensure consumer safety....

Culinary Creativity: Sprouts are versatile ingredients that can add texture and flavor to a wide range of dishes, from salads to stir-fries....

Sustainability: Sprouts are a sustainable food source, requiring fewer resources than fully grown vegetables, aligning with environmental concerns....

Personal Stories: Sprouts hold personal significance for many individuals, representing health, sustainability, culinary adventure, and cultural connections....

The Enduring Appeal...

The appeal of sprouts lies in their ability to:...

Nourish Our Bodies: Sprouts
provide essential nutrients and
health benefits that support our
well-being....

Connect Us to the Earth: Whether
grown at home or appreciated for
their sustainability, sprouts remind
us of the connection between soil,
food, and nourishment....

Inspire Culinary Creativity: The
versatility of sprouts encourages
culinary experimentation, adding
variety and excitement to our
meals....

Preserve Cultural Traditions: For
many, sprouts are a part of cultural
dishes and traditions, bridging the
gap between heritage and
modernity....

Embrace Sprouts in Your Life...

As we conclude our journey through the world of sprouts, we encourage you to embrace the versatility and nutritional benefits of sprouts in your daily life. Whether you're a health enthusiast, a sustainability advocate, a culinary explorer, or someone looking to connect with cultural roots, sprouts have something to offer....

Incorporate sprouts into your meals, experiment with new recipes, and share the enduring appeal of sprouts with friends and family. By doing so, you join a community of individuals who appreciate the unique and valuable role that sprouts play in our lives....

Thank you for joining us on this exploration of sprouts, and may your culinary adventures with sprouts continue to nourish and inspire....

Chapter 15: Sprouts - A Continuing Journey...

While we've reached the final chapter of this book, the journey with sprouts is far from over. In this concluding chapter, we'll explore the endless possibilities that lie ahead as we continue to appreciate and incorporate sprouts into our lives....

Ongoing Exploration...

The world of sprouts is vast and ever-evolving. As we move forward, there are several avenues to explore:...

New Varieties: Continually discover new types of sprouts, each with its unique flavors and textures. Experiment with lesser-known varieties and embrace the diversity of sprouts....

Innovative Recipes: Culinary creativity knows no bounds. Continue to create innovative recipes that showcase the versatility of sprouts. Share your culinary experiments with others to inspire their own kitchen adventures....

Community and Sharing: Connect with like-minded individuals who

share your passion for sprouts.
Join online communities,
participate in sprouting challenges,
and exchange tips and
experiences....

Sustainability Efforts: Explore
ways to further support sustainable
food practices in your own life.
Whether it's by growing your
sprouts at home or making
conscious choices when
purchasing food, every small
effort contributes to a greener
future....

Health and Well-being: Stay
informed about the latest research
on the health benefits of sprouts.
Consider how sprouts can
contribute to your personal

wellness goals and share this knowledge with others....

Passing the Knowledge...

As you continue your journey with sprouts, consider passing on your knowledge and experiences to the next generation. Teach your children, grandchildren, or students about the value of sprouts, both in terms of nutrition and sustainability. Inspire them to appreciate the simple joy of growing and enjoying sprouts....

The Unending Cycle...

The cycle of sprouting is a metaphor for the enduring nature of life itself. From a tiny seed, new life emerges, and with care and nourishment, it flourishes.

Sprouts remind us of the beauty and potential inherent in every small beginning....

Conclusion...

As we conclude this book, we encourage you to carry the spirit of sprouts with you on your ongoing journey. Whether you're driven by health, sustainability, culinary passion, or cultural connection, sprouts have a place in your life. Embrace their versatility, celebrate their nutritional value, and continue to explore the world of sprouts with enthusiasm....

Thank you for accompanying us on this exploration of sprouts. May your journey be filled with health, creativity, and a deeper

connection to the food you eat and
the world around you. Sprout on,
and may your life be as vibrant as
the greens that grace your plate....

www.ingramcontent.com/pod-product-compliance
Lightning Source LLC
Chambersburg PA
CBHW070753250726
48662CB00004B/1774